Aromatherapy

A Beginner's Guide To Using Aromatherapy At Home

Ruth Logan

CONTENTS

AROMATHERAPY

INTRODUCTION

Aromatherapy, also known as Essential Oil therapy, can be described as the science and art of using naturally extracted essences from plants to harmonize, balance and promote the wellbeing of the mind, body and spirit. Its aim is to unite psychological, physiological and spiritual processes to enhance the human's natural ability to heal.

It was the French perfumer and chemist, Rene- Maurice Gattefosse, who came up with the term *"aromatherapie"* in 1937 with his own publication of a book using that name. His book "Gattefosse's Aromatherapy" states his early clinical findings for making use of essential oils for a range of physiological ailments. It seems vital to understand what Gattefosse's intention for coining the word was, as he clearly meant to distinguish the medicinal application of essential oils from their perfumery applications.

So we can interpret his coining of the word *"Aromatherapie"* to mean the therapeutic application or the medicinal use of aromatic substances (essential oils) for holistic healing. But as the practice of aromatherapy has progressed, over the years, it has adopted a more holistic approach encompassing the whole body, mind and spirit (energy).

Aromatherapy is one of the oldest, ancient sciences which have been used by the doctors and some cultures of the old ages to cure ailments. The knowledge of these medicines and their practices were passed down from generation to generation and their application has become one of the major advances of natural science. Aromatherapy suggests the use of essential oils and this use of essential oils for therapeutic, spiritual, hygienic and ritualistic purposes goes back to a number of ancient civilizations who have used them in cosmetics, perfumes and drugs. It was also established by Pedanius Dioscorides, that these oils have an abundance of healing properties within them, as time goes on. This was confirmed by a French surgeon named Jean Valnet who used this technique along with other drugs to treat injured soldiers during war.

So, what does Aromatherapy suggest? It suggests that the essential oils which are found in our environment can be used to cure our ailments and increase our mental and physical wellness. These essential oils that could become a part of our daily routine could actually help and aid us in gradually removing our bodies of disease and illnesses which we have been suffering with and make us healthy. As a common man would say; the man who has his health, has his wealth intact.

This book is a guide to let you know how to practise the use of aromatherapy at home. In this book you will find everything you need to know to get your feet wet and discover the uses of essential oils in aromatherapy, for yourself and your home. But please remember that you need to be responsible when sourcing the oils for these ingredients, as stated in the book, from reliable manufacturers.

There are unlimited ways in which these oils can be used but moderation is key because a little can go a long way. The benefits and applications of the different types of recipes are given below as well, to give you an insight of how to use them and a taster into what is out there.

In some places of worship the techniques used to relax the mind and be stress-free are based around aromatherapy and in many organic products, essential oils have taken the place of many fragrances and other harsh chemicals. These oils are perfect to make a perfume because of their long lasting consistency and their ability to take you into a relaxed state of mind. This is why aromatherapy is also commonplace amongst people who meditate.

Now, let us dive into this wonderful world of aromatherapy, its uses, practices, and how well and efficiently you can apply it into your own life.

CHAPTER 1: AROMATHERAPY – BASICS

What Is Aromatherapy?

Aromatherapy is the process of using natural materials to improve a person's mental or physical state. The practice, which now is known popularly as a form of alternative medicine, began hundreds of years ago within previous civilizations in Egypt, China, and Greece, and was used for both therapeutic and ceremonial purposes. The materials used in aromatherapy are various natural oils taken from parts of plants or trees. In spite of its early usage, the term aromatherapy was not introduced until the early 1900s by European scientists when it was first used to heal wounds during World War II.

The definition of aromatherapy can be viewed in different perspectives, as is known as a method to heal mainly through smell and how it can interact with ones emotions. However, this can be untrue. Each essential oil has a different effect on our bodies natural chemistry causes an effect mentally, physically, and emotionally. For example, any type of product you put on your body is easily absorbed through your skin and therefore into your body. In this book, various uses will be demonstrated on how essential oils can be applied topically on certain areas of your body depending on your current issue to relieve any pain. This shows how concentrated these oils are, and how they absorb through your body at different levels.

Aromatherapy, as you may know, can be considered as a form of herbal medicine, as essential oils can be applied and prepared in various ways with a botanical context.

How Aromatherapy Works

Aromatherapy is practiced using three main methods, each having its own distinct advantages. The first is known as aerial diffusion, which is followed by dispersing a select mixture within the air in order to both clean and enhance the user's breathing experience. The second is direct inhaling. Much as the name implies, this method is less concerned with the surrounding atmosphere and focuses more on immediate ingestion. The third method is topical application which is carried out through direct contact with the skin. Selecting which method to use greatly depends on both the intent of treatment and a user's personal preference.

The materials used within the practice of aromatherapy are numerous and in a state of constant growth as humanity gains more understanding of the natural world around it. In general, aroma therapists make use of the following sources:

Essential oils, also referred to as natural oils, are extracted from various parts of the plant such as its leaves or roots through the use of steam distillation. The end result is a highly concentrated, aromatic liquid which can be used for different purposes such as aromatherapy. Other uses include making soaps, flavoring foods, or the production of perfumes. Examples of popular essential oils used today are peppermint, eucalyptus, and tea tree oil. The top ones to choose as a staple in your home includes tea tree, lemon, peppermint, lavender, eucalyptus, and arnica.

Absolutes are also extracted from plants. Unlike essential oils, chemicals are required in the process of obtaining them from natural ingredients. Absolutes are often obtained from specific plants when the use of steam is not capable of extracting essential oils. The process of using chemical solvents for extraction often results in a more concentrated final product but does leave small traces of residual chemicals behind. Absolutes are very popular in the production of perfumes. Examples of absolutes include blue lily, jasmine, and vanilla.

Carrier oils are used in order to reduce the concentration of the essential oils or absolutes used within aromatherapy. This is a vital step before applying essential oils directly to the body. There is a wide range of carrier oils in use, including popular choices such as olive oil and peanut oil. The choice of carrier oil depends on its intended usage and the different essential oils or absolutes it will be paired with. Carrier oils in general are easy to find and fairly inexpensive. Carrier oils are common in recipes for children, as essential oils should be diluted prior to applying to the skin to avoid irritation and any sensitivity. Some common carrier oils include sweet almond oil, sunflower oil, coconut oil, or even jojoba oil.

Herbal distillates are gathered similarly to essential oils. When essential oils are steam distilled, there is also a watery distillate left behind. This byproduct is the herbal distillate and is useful in many aroma therapeutic practices. A popular example is rose water.

Infused oils are carrier oils which have been, as the name infers, infused with further additives. These additives are often different herbs. Infused oils can then be used instead of carrier oils and have the added advantage of the herbs they contain. Infused oils are easy to make and have seen increased popularity as aromatherapy continues to become a more accepted household practice.

Phytoncides are organic compounds produced from plants. Phytoncides are produced by plants such as; onions and different varieties of trees. In nature, these compounds work to keep the plant alive by preventing decay and attack from outside animals. As human knowledge has advanced, they have become more and more common in medicinal usages such as aromatherapy.

Along with the many types of materials used, there is a wide range of benefits within the realm of aromatherapy. Different sources list varying benefits that are both cognitive and physical. The following health benefits have been reported through various methods of aromatherapy:

Stress relief is often listed as the most common usage of aromatherapy. Stress is a common response from the brain when a person is placed under great demand, change, or intense situations. As the current culture becomes increasingly fast paced, there has been a large outpour of available pharmaceutical medications, self-help books, and counseling made available for the sole purpose of dealing with stress. Aromatherapy provides another outlet to everyday people for dealing with the stress of everyday life. Because certain methods of aromatherapy are low cost and materials are highly accessible, the rise in stress in recent history has had a large impact on the greater usage of aromatherapy. Along similar lines, aromatherapy has shown a capacity to reduce depression. Scent can have a powerful impact on a person's overall disposition or mood.

Memory has also been reported as an area of improvement from aromatherapy. Certain combinations have shown a positive effect on both increased short term memory, as well as an ability to slow the process of memory loss. Aromatherapy has become a popular option for those struggling with dementia, and thus is an option which should be considered as older relatives and friends begin to show signs of memory loss.

As a form of alternative medicine, specific essential oils and methods of aromatherapy have shown signs of improving the human body's ability to *heal or recover* from certain types of injuries or sicknesses. This is thought to be due to essential oils' anti-microbial properties along with certain scents' ability to improve oxygen intake.

Similar to aromatherapy's ability to reduce depression and stress levels is its ability to *increase energy levels*. In today's culture where unhealthy high caffeine options are found in abundance, aromatherapy provides a beneficial alternative. Aromatherapy is obviously not the only healthy life choice required in order to feel rested and awake throughout the day, but it is a possible positive contributor to raised energy levels and increased cognitive activity.

Riding the coat tails of the above benefit is aromatherapy's ability to improve a person's overall *sleep*. The use of aromatherapy can not only decrease the dependence on caffeine infused beverages which can result in difficulty falling asleep, but it has also shown an ability to improve the body's ability to stay on a more natural sleep cycle. Various natural oils even have varying sedative effects.

Aromatherapy has shown strong correlations with its ability to *relieve pain*, most notably headaches. Reduced headaches come from natural oils' ability to reduce stress, as discussed earlier, along with an ability to work as a form of anesthesia within the body.

As a form of preventative medicine, aromatherapy is also thought to positively improve a person's *immune system*. Once again, this correlation is thought to be highly dependent on the oil's anti-microbial effects.

For each of these potential benefits from aromatherapy, there are specific essential oils which work best. Determining which essential oils and materials to use should be dependent on specific aroma therapeutic goals and researched by reading further in this book.

A lot of research has been done within aromatherapy, and the results are not always clear. For such reasons, aromatherapy has been labeled as an alternative form of medicine. All of this means is that it is a form of healing which does not originate from direct use of the scientific method. Other popular forms of alternative medicine include chiropractic medicine and acupuncture. While aromatherapy might not be clinical, there is no denying its positive effects on the human body when used appropriately. Generally, aromatherapy is thought to work by using specific scents to send messages to your brain through communication with the nose. Different areas of the brain can be stimulated through inhaling essential oils resulting in both mental and physical influences. Similar concepts hold true when aromatherapy is practiced through direct skin contact or aroma therapeutic massage.

The heritage of aromatherapy started locally, within families and towns with access to the plants and natural resources required. With the rapid urbanization of the 1900s within the developed world, practices such as aromatherapy became a luxury for much of the world. In high density cities, ingredients such as essential oils and plant materials are by obvious inspection more scarce. Thanks in great part to advanced internet commerce and rapid distribution systems available today, the practice of aromatherapy is accessible to a high percentage of the population. In addition, the explosion of available knowledge through the internet coupled with an increasing social awareness and desire to retreat from the chemical and clinical solutions of previous generations has made the term 'aromatherapy' a household word. In short, it is a great time to begin practicing aromatherapy.

How To Use Aromatherapy At Home?

There are many resources to begin practicing aromatherapy within one's own home and the following chapters of this book will attempt to give the reader helpful, practical information about entering into healthy aroma therapeutic practices. These aromatherapy practices will span the three main categories of common ailments, household applications and general beauty.

Users should always take precaution in being highly informed about the materials and methods they use for either inhalation or topical application. Aromatherapy has great beneficial effects, but anything taken into the body at incorrect concentrations can be unhealthy. Along with this, each essential oil has a different property that can interact with your body. Therefore, before using an essential oil take into account the person's age, health, and so forth. It is important to research what common uses each one is used for, as they all provide different reactions to your body. Always take precautions when taking them internally, and avoid direct contact to your eyes. Always buy ingredients that are pure and natural, and if pre-blended ensure that these ingredients are natural as well.

Aromatherapy at home provides many benefits; first being not having to purchase common household products at the store. This includes making your own diffuser, lotions, body washes, pain reliever, and even beauty products such as lip gloss. Following chapters will give readers a look at appropriate aroma therapeutic practices for their own home and daily lives along with insight on the proper use for each ailment.

CHAPTER 2: AROMATHERAPY FOR COMMON AILMENTS

Using aromatic plants to treat common ailments can be dated back to 3000 BC. Before modern medicine, all the medicine came straight from plant sources. In fact may have been more widely and successfully used to treat common ailments throughout history than they are today.

The essential oils used in aromatherapy are derived from plants and enter the body through inhalation, direct application to skin, bloodstream or ingested. It is not recommended that the later application of ingesting aromatherapy be done at home, please consult a professional if you wish to use aromatherapy internally.

Many common ailments symptoms can be relieved or altogether prevented with the use of aromatherapy at home. By altering brain function or entering the blood stream, the essential oils used can greatly affect how you feel and can relieve common ailments.

Be sure to purchase high quality pure essential oils as the prices can vary with the quality of the oils, you generally get what you pay for and the effects might not be as strong with poorer quality oils.

Always be careful when using aromatherapy with children. There are some essential oils that are not suitable for children and others that need to be diluted with a carrier oil before they are administered. Essential oils may also affect pregnant woman differently or should not be used at all when pregnant.

A carrier oil is a vegetable based oil derived from fats (such as olive oil, coconut oil, jojoba oil and grapeseed oil) that are used to dilute the essential oils that are known to cause skin irritation when applied in their pure forms.

Arthritis

Finding relief from pain and inflammation caused by arthritis can be difficult, but it can be done at home with aromatherapy. The best way to use aromatherapy for arthritis is to take a bath in certain essential oils or massaging a blend of oils directly onto sore joints.

The best essential oils for arthritis are the oils that are high in linalool and linalyl acetate as they are shown to have anti-inflammatory and pain relieving components. Two essential oils with high linalool and linalyl acetate are lavender and bergamot.

Other essential oils that have been proven to help with arthritis are; eucalyptus, orange, peppermint, German chamomile, rosemary, marjoram and ginger.

Soaking in a warm bath for 20 – 30 minutes can be beneficial for arthritis suffers and when you add in essential oils, you'll feel much better. Try this recipe for your next warm bath.

Arthritis Relief Bath Soak:

- Juniper berry essential oil – 4 drops
- Cypress essential oil – 2 drops
- Rosemary essential oil – 2 drop
- Lavender essential oil – 2 drops
- Bath salts – 1-2 cups (mix equal parts baking soda with Epsom salts)

Add the oils to the bath while it is running or just when the tub is full. Soak in the bath for 20 – 30 minutes.

Massaging essential oils into your joints in need of attention can also greatly reduce your pain and inflammation. Try these two recipes when you feel swollen and in need of relief.

Arthritis Anti-Inflammatory Blend:

- German Chamomile – 5 drops

- Geranium – 4 drops

- Yellow Birch – 4 drops

- Rosemary – 3 drops

- Grapeseed oil – 30 ml

Mix the oils together in a dark glass jar, shaking well before each application. Massage swollen joints with the blend, daily if needed. Do not apply to broken skin.

Arthritis Warming Pain Relief Blend:

- Roman Chamomile – 6 drops

- Marjoram – 4 drops

- Coriander – 3 drops

- Rosemary – 3 drops

- Vanilla Blend – 2 drops

- Black Pepper – 1 drop

- Ginger – 1 drop

- Carrier oil (of your choice) – 10 drops

Blend all the oils into a dark glass jar, shaking well before use. Do not apply to broken skin. Massage in joints that require pain relief.

Coughs

Many times a coughing fit comes on in the middle of the night when you do not want to leave the house and the stores are closed. Using aromatherapy can greatly reduce coughs right at home. Aromatherapy uses essential oils to relieve coughing in two ways, through inhaling the fumes of the oil or by rubbing the oil onto your chest.

There are a few different ways you can inhale essential oils to relieve coughing symptoms. One way is to drop the essential oils into a bowl of steaming water. Place your head a few inches from the bowl with a towel draped over your head so you are inhaling the fumes. You can also soak a cloth in the oils and place it in front of your mouth to inhale.

Another way to inhale the essential oils is to use a Terra Cotta Disc, a passive type diffuser, in the shower. Place the oils in the diffuser and place the diffuser on the shower floor so that the warm water hits the diffuser to dispense the oils. You can also use a fan diffuser to dispense the oils at night placing it next to your bed.

To rub the essential oils onto your chest, always use a carrier oil so the oils do not irritate your skin.

The best essential oils to relieve coughing are: eucalyptus, peppermint, thieves blend, basil, frankincense, silver fir, sandalwood, cedarwood, tea tree, thyme, myrrh and cajeput.

Cough Relieving Steam Blend:

- Eucalyptus – 3 drops
- Basil – 3 drops
- Frankincense – 3 drops
- Silver Fir – 3 drops
- Peppermint – 3 drops

Using a bowl of almost boiled water, drop the oils into the bowl. Place your head over the bowl with a towel over your head to trap the vapours. Breathe deeply for a few minutes until you start to feel relief.

Cough Relieving Aromatherapy Rub:

- Eucalyptus – 12 drops

- Peppermint – 5 drops

- Thyme – 5 drops

- Olive Oil – 5 drops

Mix the ingredients in a dark glass jar, shaking well before use. Rub mixture onto chest and throat as needed, especially before bed.

Natural Cough Syrup:

- Lemon – 1 Drop

- Orange – 1 drop

- Frankincense – 1 drop

- Peppermint – 1 drop

- Honey – 1 tsp

Add all of these ingredients onto a spoon or a vodka glass and swallow.

Eczema

People who suffer from eczema know how difficult it is to treat the symptoms. Often over the counter lotions are not enough to reduce the itchy inflamed skin. There are several essential oils that can great reduce the symptoms of your eczema and possibly eliminate the eczema altogether.

Some of the best essential oils for soothing the itching, pain and inflammation from eczema are: German chamomile, yarrow, helichrysum, lavender, calendula and geranium. These oils are particularly beneficial because they are anti-inflammatory, skin rejuvenators, anti-bacterial, moisturizing and/or pain and itch reliving.

Aromatherapy for eczema can be applied in several different ways. You can make your own eczema moisturizing lotion, use the oils in a skin-cooling compress, take a soothing bath in specific essential oils or make a skin-cooling spray. Use the following recipes for each different application method.

Eczema Aromatherapy Moisturizer:

- Lavender – 2 drops
- Helichrysum – 1 drop
- German chamomile OR yarrow – 1 drop
- Carrier oil – 5 tbsp

Combine all the ingredients together in an airtight container, mixing well. Apply to eczema in the morning and at night, after a warm bath is best to make sure the skin is clean and the moisture stays locked in.

Eczema Essential Oil Compress:

- Lavender – 2 drops
- German chamomile – 2 drops
- Geranium – 1 drop
- ½ cup cold water

Put all the ingredients into a shallow bowl and stir. Place a clean cloth on the surface of the water to get all the oils. Apply the compress to inflamed skin.

Eczema Relieving Bath:

- Sandalwood – 4 drops

- Chamomile – 4 drops

- Tea Tree Oil – 4 drops

- Jojoba Oil – 6 tbsp

Mix all the ingredients together in a dark glass container. After you have run a warm bath, place 2 tablespoons of the mixture into your bath and soak in the tub for 20 – 30 minutes. The jojoba oil acts as a carrier oil and will help moisturize.

Skin-Cooling Lavender Spray:

- Lavender – 13 drops

- ½ cup distilled water

- Spray bottle

Mix the lavender and water into the spray bottle, shaking before use. Spray onto eczema affected areas.

Fatigue

Ever felt drained and over tired? We all have. Some of us suffer from fatigue more than others, but there are a few aromatherapy tricks to help pick you up and give you the energy boost you need. Chronic fatigue can be caused by a number of reasons and you should consult your health professional to find the root cause. Short-term fatigue can be aided by aromatherapy; however, only rest can truly reset your body. Long-term exhaustion can be a more serious health problem.

Essential oils can be great for helping your brain function and giving you the energy you need to go about your day. They can be used as a massage oil, inhaled, put into a diffuser to dispense into a room or used as a perfume to smell as needed.

One of the fastest ways to reduce fatigue is by increasing blood flow in your brain. Rosemary has shown to do just that. Inhale a few deep breaths of rosemary essential oil out of the bottle and you'll have increased cerebral blood flow. However, due to its effectiveness, do not inhale rosemary within 6 hours of going to sleep, as you could be awake longer than you planned to be.

The oils to wake you up are: basil, cloves, peppermint, orange, black pepper, cinnamon, eucalyptus, lemon and rosemary. These oils do a better job than a cup of coffee.

Pick Me Up Aromatherapy:

- Lemon – 8 drops

- Eucalyptus – 2 drops

- Peppermint – 2 drops

- Cinnamon Leaf – 1 drop

- Cardamom – 1 drop

- Carrier oil – 2 tbsp

Combine all these oils into a dark glass container. Shake before use. This combination can be used as a massage oil, used as a perfume put onto your wrists or temples, or put 2 tablespoons into a bath and soak for 20 – 30 minutes. If you want to use this combination in a diffuser simply do not put in the carrier oil.

Stimulating Aromatherapy Blend:

- Orange – 3 drops

- Clary Sage – 2 drops

- Coriander – 2 drops

- Helichrysum – 1 drop

- Jasmine – 1 drop

- Palmarosa – 1 drop

- Vetiver – 1 drop

- Jojoba Oil – 2 tbsp

Mix all the oils together and use as a perfume or inhale from an inhaler or a few drops on tissue. You can also omit the jojoba oil and use as a diffuser in a room.

Fever

Having a fever is sometimes a good thing; it means your body is fighting off the foreign invaders that are trying to take over your body. But having a fever is never fun. There are some easy ways to use aromatherapy at home to reduce your fever or possibly make it disappear completely.

The most simple and effective way is to massage a couple of drops of pure peppermint oil onto the bottoms of your feet and back of your neck. However, if you are trying to lower the fever of a small child, then use a carrier oil to dilute the peppermint oil or replace it completely with lavender oil.

Other essentials oils that can be used to treat fevers are: bergamot, eucalyptus, black pepper, ginger, lemon, chamomile, sandalwood and tea tree.

Using these oils as a body massage should be avoided if you have a fever. Instead they should be applied through a cold compress, inhaled via steam or in a room diffuser. Aromatherapy for fevers will only work if the fever is mild. For severe fevers, especially in children, see a health care professional.

Fever Reducer:

- 5 drops Pure Peppermint Essential oil

- 1 Tbsp Organic, unrefined Coconut Oil

Mix the peppermint oil and coconut oil together. Apply to the bottom of the feet and back of the net, you may also apply a cool ice pack on the back of the neck after applying the oils. Apply this recipe to the specified areas every 15 minutes.

Feel Better Today Recipe:

- 5 drops of Frankincense

- 6 drops of Oregano

- 5 drops of Lemon

- 5 drops of Thieves

Mix the ingredients together and apply them in a roller bottle, while adding carrier oil like coconut oil to fill the remaining bottle. You can apply this to your feet and the back of your neck. If you do not have a roller bottle, you may apply this as you normally would to your neck and feet, or to a diffuser that is near you.

Eucalyptus Cooler:

- 3-5 drops of Pure Peppermint essential oil

- 3-5 drops of Eucalyptus essential oil

- 3-5 drops of Thieves essential oil

Mix the above essential oils and apply to these areas at least three to four times daily until the fever subsides: upper back, chest, back of neck, and forehead. Ensure you keep away from your eyes.

Headaches

Aromatherapy is very effective at alleviating headache pain. The essential oils can be used as a massage oil, in a diffuser, as a compress or inhaled to help relax your muscles and relieve headache pain.

The best essential oil for almost every type of headache is peppermint, followed by rosemary, lavender, eucalyptus, jasmine and helichrysum.

Mix 1 ounce of carrier oil, such as sweet almond or jojoba, with 10 drops of any of the essential oils listed above (8 drops if using peppermint or eucalyptus) to create a massage oil to soothe headaches. Using a few drops, massage the oil onto your forehead, back of the neck, temples, scalp and shoulders.

You can also put a combination of these essential oils into a diffuser to use aromatically in a room while you are resting. Or drop the oils of your choosing onto cotton balls to smell as needed while you have a headache.

To use a cold compress to relieve your headache, use 1 cup of cold water with 5 drops of lavender or eucalyptus. Apply the compress to your forehead and repeat as often as necessary.

Headache Be-Gone Aromatherapy Recipe:

- Peppermint – 20 drops
- Eucalyptus – 17 drops
- Cajeput – 15 drops
- Rosemary – 10 drops
- Lavender – 10 drops
- Helichrysum – 1 drop
- Carrier oil of your choice – 10 drops

Mix all the oils together. If you have a roll on glass bottle, use that to mix and apply the mixture to your forehead and temples. If you do not have a glass bottle, simply massage the mixed oils onto your forehead and temples.

Sinus Headache Recipe:

- 2 drops Frankincense Essential Oil
- 2 drops Lavender Essential Oil
- 2 drops Peppermint Essential oil
- 1 tsp coconut oil

Blend together the above ingredients; apply to sinus areas such as the centre of your forehead and your temple areas. Ensure you are careful around your eyes.

Relieving Headache & Sinus Pressure:

- 8 drops of Eucalyptus Essential Oil
- 4 drops of Peppermint Essential Oil

Blend together the above ingredients. Similar to the blend above, apply to areas of pain such as your temples, back of neck, and forehead. Be cautious around your eyes.

Headache Reliever Roll on Recipe:

- 10 drops Lavender Essential Oil
- 6 Drops Peppermint Essential Oil
- 5 Drops Frankincense Essential Oil
- Fill remaining of the bottle with Organic Coconut Oil

This recipe is perfect for on the go, always available, headache reliever. Apply to areas of pain, and as always, try to avoid sensitive areas like your eyes.

Insomnia

In today's society insomnia has become a problem for many people. With the busy lives we lead, it can be difficult to settle down and sleep at night. While aromatherapy for insomnia does not come to mind as a solution right away, it has been found to help fight insomnia.

There are several essential oils that are known to help relax your body and soothe your mind. These oils will make all your distractions disappear so you can prepare to get a proper nights' sleep.

To calm and relax you the best essentials oils are: lavender, jasmine, chamomile, ylang ylang, marjoram, sweet orange and rose.

The best use of these essential oils to fight insomnia is to draw a warm bath and drop in 5 drops of your favourite oils listed above before you go to bed. Alternatively you can drop a few drops onto a piece of tissue and put the tissue inside your pillowcase (just be sure to change the tissue each night). You can also place 3 drops of each oil that you like into a diffuser next to your bed at night. Or make a massage oil blend of the oils mixed with a carrier oil to apply the oils directly to your skin.

Use the following recipe without the carrier oil to use in a bath, on a tissue or in a diffuser to help get rid of your insomnia. With the carrier oil it can be used as a massage oil to help really relax all your muscles.

Insomnia Aromatherapy Blend:

- Lavender – 2 drops
- Geranium – 2 drops
- Sweet Orange – 1 drop
- Roman chamomile – 1 drop
- Carrier oil of your choice – 10 ml

Mix all the oils together in a dark glass jar. Shake gently before each application.

If you are trying to relax before bed, there are some essential oils that act as stimulants and you should avoid them. Some stimulating essential oils are: peppermint, lemon, rosemary, grapefruit and cypress. These are much better at fighting fatigue than insomnia.

A Good Night's Sleep:

- 5 drops Lavender Essential Oil

- 7 drops Roman Chamomile

A good nights rest involves going to bed relaxed, and ready to go to sleep. Adding these ingredients to a diffuser by your bed will help you relax and breathe in the mixture as you lay there. You may also apply the mixture to the back of your neck and your chest to take in the full benefits.

Bedtime Routine:

- 1 tbsp Organic Coconut Oil

- 5 drops Lavender Essential Oil

- 5 drops Cedarwood Essential Oil

- 4 drops Roman Chamomile Essential Oil

This recipe can be a bedtime routine that is worth getting used to. Apply this to your chest and neck prior to lying down. It is important before bed to practice mindful breathing to take in the full experience of how essential oils can help your bedtime routine and promote sleep.

Menopause

Menopause has all sorts of physical, mental and emotional effects on your body. Since aromatherapy has an effect on how the brain functions, it can greatly help relieve symptoms of menopause. Aromatherapy can help balance your emotional equilibrium and reduce hot flashes.

Clary sage is the best essential oil to treat menopause. It is great for hot flashes, night sweats, insomnia and helps to balance hormones. It is a fairly potent oil, so not much is needed. Geranium is also an important essential oil in balancing hormones.

To maximize your aromatherapy for menopause, use clary sage, geranium, Roman chamomile, neroli, lemon, yarrow, rose, lavender, ylang ylang and jasmine.

These oils can be used in a diffuser, as a spray or as a massage oil when mixed with a carrier oil, in a warm bath, inhaled from a tissue or cotton ball or a used as a compress.

Getting right to the point, the most common issue with menopause are the hot flashes. You can use the following recipe in any of the application methods listed above to relieve your hot flashes whenever they hit.

Hot Flashes Be Gone Aromatherapy:

- Clary Sage – 10 drops
- Geranium – 11 drops
- Lemon – 7 drops
- Sage – 2 drops
- For massage oil – 30 ml of carrier oil

Mix the essential oils together to be used in the bath, inhaled from a tissue, for a compress with water or in a spray bottle with water. To make a massage oil, combine the essential oils with the carrier oil.

Menopause Daily Body Oil/Lotion:

- Lemon – 6 drops

- Geranium – 5 drops

- Clary Sage – 2 drops

- Angelica – 1 drop

- Jasmine – 1 drop

- Carrier oil or unscented lotion – 10 drops

Mix everything together in a dark glass bottle and use at least once a day as a body oil/lotion or add 1 tablespoon to your bath. If you prefer a creamier lotion then use the lotion instead of the oil.

Menstrual Cramps

Menstrual cramps can be insufferable for some women, causing them fall over from the pain or not leave their bed for the duration of their period. Luckily there is hope and proven pain relief from aromatherapy. Some essential oils such as clary sage and sweet fennel have shown to regulate menstrual cycles.

The essential oils can help to soothe and relax you, improving your mood and irritability. Other oils will help to relieve pain, acting as local anaesthetics and helping to dilate blood vessels and therefore reduce cramping.

Essential oils that have been proven to relieve pain from menstrual cramps are: lavender, clary sage, rose, marjoram, German chamomile and sweet fennel. To best use the essential oils to reduce menstrual cramps are to use them as a massage oil, a compress or in a warm bath.

Menstrual Cramp Oil Blend:

- Clary Sage – 20 drops
- Sweet Marjoram – 20 drops
- German Chamomile – 15 drops
- Rose – 10 drops
- Carrier oil of your choice – 20 drops

Mix all the oils into a dark glass jar, shake gently before each application. If using the menstrual cramp oil blend in a warm bath, then use 2 teaspoons added to the bath water and soak for 20 – 30 minutes. For a compress use 10 drops of the mixture in hot water, placing a cloth on the water then onto your abdomen. To use as a massage oil, use a couple of drops of the mixture and massage your lower abdomen and lower back.

Menstrual Cramp Massage Oils:

- Lavender – 4 drops
- Clary Sage – 2 drops
- Rose – 2 drops
- Almond or Olive Oil – 5 drops

Mix all the oils together and massage onto lower abdomen and lower back in a clockwise motion as needed to alleviate menstrual cramps.

Migraines

Migraines differ from headaches in that they can have other symptoms throughout the body and they tend to have more severe pain than the typical headaches. Migraines can be accompanied by sensitivity to light, nausea, vomiting, throbbing, seeing auras around objects and often is on just one side of the head.

Migraines often completely incapacitate their sufferers. If you suffer from migraines you know the severity of pain associated with them and that over the counter medications sometimes do not help reduce the pain.

Aromatherapy can greatly reduce the pain associated with migraines as well as ease nausea. The essential oils used to relieve migraines are very similar to relieving the pain from headaches. The best oils to use are: peppermint, sandalwood, lavender, eucalyptus, rosemary, jasmine and sweet marjoram.

Essential oils can be used in several ways to treat migraines. They can be used as smelling salts, as a massage oil or roll on, in a diffuser or a compress. Sweet marjoram can be used as a hot or cold compress on the back of the neck to improve blood flow to your brain.

Migraine Relieving Smelling Salts:

- Small dark glass bottle (clean and empty essential oil bottle)

- Dead Sea Salt

- Fractionated Coconut Oil to fill glass bottle 75%

- Peppermint oil – 6 drops

- Lemongrass – 4 drops

- Sandalwood – 2 drops

- Eucalyptus – 2 drops

Fill the bottle with Dead Sea salt. Then fill the bottle about 75% with the fractionated coconut oil and add the essential oils. Put on the cap and shake the bottle gently. Smell as needed for migraine pain relief.

Quick Migraine Relief Massage Oil:

- Peppermint – 6 drops
- Eucalyptus – 4 drops
- Myrrh – 2 drops
- Almond Oil – 5 drops

Mix all the oils together and massage into your forehead, temples and back of your neck.

Headache Helper Roll-on:

- Peppermint – 10 drops
- Lavender – 6 drops
- Frankincense – 5 drops
- Fractionated Coconut Oil – 8.5 ml
- Roller bottle – 10 ml

Fill the 10ml bottle with the essential oils first and then the carrier oil, secure with the roller top and shake well. Massage onto temples and anywhere else where it's tight.

Muscle Soreness

Your muscles may be sore for a number of reasons, including illness, cramping, fatigue, spasms, sprains or tension. Muscles are most commonly sore from working out and not stretching properly before or after the work out causing muscles to tighten, inflame and cramp.

Essential oils can be help in reducing muscle soreness by reducing inflammation, relaxing the muscles by sedating your nervous system and muscles and easing pain. To get the full effects from aromatherapy to reduce muscle soreness, the oils are applied topically to the sore muscles through massaging and cold presses or used in a warm bath. The motion of massaging muscles combined with the essential oils will be the most beneficial way to reduce muscle soreness with aromatherapy.

The best essential oils to reduce muscle pain are: marjoram, rosemary, peppermint, basil, cypress, ginger, lavender, wintergreen, lemongrass, birch, rosemary, chamomile, jasmine and white fir.

Marjoram has sedative properties while rosemary has antispasmodic and anti-inflammatory properties; both of which are great for reducing muscle soreness. Lavender will relax muscles and chamomile will reduce swelling.

Aromatherapy Muscle Pain Relief Oil:

- Lavender – 12 drops
- Marjoram – 6 drops
- Chamomile – 4 drops
- Ginger – 4 drops
- Carrier Oil or St. John's Wort – 10 drops

Mix all the ingredients together in a dark glass jar, shaking gently before each application. To use massage onto the sore muscle as needed throughout the day.

Lavender Muscle Relaxing Aromatherapy Bath:

- Lavender – 10 drops
- Frankincense – 5 drops
- Marjoram – 5 drops
- Cedarwood – 1 drop
- Carrier Oil – 20 drops

Mix all the oils into a small dark glass bottle. When you are ready to relieve your aching muscles, pour one tablespoon of the mixture into your bath water right after it has finished filling. Soak for 20 – 30 minutes.

Muscle Strain Healer:

- Basil – 4 drops

- Clove – 3 drops

- Eucalyptus – 4 drops

- Lavender – 6 drops

- Marjoram – 3 drops

- Rosemary – 4 drops

- Grapeseed oil – 6 tsp

Mix essential oils and carrier oils together in a small bowl and slowly massage into sore muscles and other tight or strained areas.

Nausea

Everyone has had nausea at one point in his or her life. It's not pleasant and has a large variety of causes from motion sickness to anxiety to food poisoning to pregnancy to bad smells and everything else in between.

Aromatherapy can provide quick relief to a nauseated stomach. Since nausea can be caused by poor smells, it can be remedied with pleasant smells in the form of specific essential oils such as peppermint and ginger. The quickest ways for these oils to work is by inhaling a drop or two on a tissue or cotton ball, or in an inhaler, or just open the bottle of the ginger or peppermint oil and smell.

Other essential oils that work well to alleviate nausea are: cardamom, fennel, lavender, basil, coriander and for some people Roman Chamomile.

All Purpose Nausea Relief Abdominal Oil:

- Lemongrass – 2 drops

- Chamomile – 2 drops

- Ginger – 2 drops

- Fennel – 1 drop

- Cardamom – 1 drop

- Carrier oil of your choice – 10 drops

You can use any carrier oil you like. Mix all the oils together in a dark glass bottle. Massage the oil onto your abdomen in a clockwise motion to relieve nausea symptoms from gas, indigestion, motion sickness, stress and anxiety. You can also use this recipe in a warm bath.

Aromatherapy to Eliminate Nausea and Vomiting:

- Basil – 1 drop

- Lavender – 1 drop

- Peppermint – 1 drop

- Carrier oil of your choice – 2 tbsp

Mix the oils together and use immediately. Put the oil in your hands and rub them together to warm the oil. Massage the oil in a clockwise direction on your abdomen. When finished, cup hands in front of your mouth and nose and inhale a few slow deep breaths.

If you are prone to motion sickness, then you can use aromatherapy as a preventive measure before you get into your vehicle and during the trip. Simply inhale any of the aforementioned essential oils 30 – 60 minutes before you leave for the trip and every 15 – 30 minutes during the trip. If it's too late and motion sickness has already set in then try the following recipe.

Aromatherapy for Motion Sickness:

- Roman Chamomile – 10 drops

- Peppermint – 10 drops

- Ginger – 10 drops

Mix the oils in a dark bottle and inhale a few deep breaths every 15 – 30 minutes until the nausea subsides.

Rashes

Rashes on your skin can be uncomfortable, itchy, painful and sometimes embarrassing. Rashes can be caused by any number of things and sometimes you'll never really know what caused the rash in the first place. Rashes can be caused by allergic reactions from something ingested, they can be from nutritional deficiencies, viral or fungal infections, parasites and medications.

While you are figuring out the cause of your rash to treat it at the cause, you can use essential oils to help reduce the itching and redness. The best essential oils for reducing rashes are: lavender, chamomile, tea tree, cedar wood, peppermint, helichrysum, patchouli, sandalwood, frankincense and geranium.

For a baby with a diaper rash, it is best to use diluted lavender or chamomile oil and apply it directly to the rash. Or you can add 2 drops to the baby's bath water. This can also be applied to a rash for adults.

All aromatherapy for rashes are best used when applied topically, directly to the rash or in a warm bath where the oils can come in contact with the skin. To soothe inflamed and itching skin you can try the following recipe to reduce the inflammation ease the pain and stop the itching.

Anti-Itching Aromatherapy Recipe:

- Lavender – 5 drops

- Frankincense – 5 drops

- Tea Tree – 3 drops

- Witch Hazel to fill small glass bottle

In a small glass bottle, add the essential oils and then fill the bottle with witch hazel. This recipe is good to apply to heat rashes, bug bits, poison ivy, hives, allergic reactions and anything that causes itching. Tea tree oil is anti-fungal and anti-bacterial, lavender is pain relieving, frankincense helps with cell rejuvenation and the witch hazel is naturally soothing and is an astringent.

If you suffer from rosacea, this recipe will reduce the redness and rash using a spray.

Rosacea Calming Spray:

- Oregano – 8 drops

- Lavender – 5 drops

- Tea Tree – 5 drops

- Apple Cider Vinegar – 1 oz

- Natural Aloe Vera Gel – 1 oz

Mix the apple cider vinegar and aloe vera gel together first in a small spray bottle. Add the essential oils and shake. Closing your eyes and being very careful not to get any of the mixture in your eyes, spray the mixture directly onto your rosacea. This can also be used on other rashes as well.

Stress

Stress is likely the most common culprit for the things that ail us. Stress can be caused by a variety of things and sometimes we do not even realize we are stressed out before our bodies remind us. Daily life can wear us down and affect us in ways we do not even realize.

Using aromatherapy on a daily basis to reduce stress should be in everyone's daily routine. It can greatly improve your day to day life by making you feel more relaxed and able to conquer anything that comes your way. Aromatherapy for stress is possibly the most common use for aromatherapy.

You can use aromatherapy as a preventative measure or if you are feeling particularly stressed out, then aromatherapy can help you to calm down. The best application for aromatherapy for stress relief is to use a diffuser in a room so that the oils are dispensed in the air and you do not have to worry about attending to them. A diffuser is the best stress preventing application of aromatherapy.

Other ways to de-stress using aromatherapy is to use essential oils in a warm bath or having someone give you an essential oil massage. This will greatly help to calm you down and relax your body and mind. Taking the time out of your day to focus on yourself with the essential oils will improve your overall well-being.

The best stress relieving essential oils are; rose, lavender, bergamont, frankinscense, vanilla, marjoram, vetvier, sandalwood, German chamomile and ylang ylang.

Stress Relieving Massage Oil:

- Lavender – 12 drops

- Bergamont – 12 drops

- Marjoram – 3 drops

- Clary Sage – 2 drops

- Vetvier – 1 drop

- Carrier oil of your choice – 20 drops

Mix all the oils in a dark glass bottle, at least 24 hours before you want to use them so that the oils have time to cure. The bottle can be stored in a cool, dark place for up to 3 months. Using a little at a time, use as a massage oil and feel the stress disappear. If you are alone, give yourself a foot massage, rub on your temples, chest and stomach. If you have someone to help, get them to give you a full body massage.

Relaxing 'Woodsy' Diffuser Blend:

- Lavender – 4 drops

- Cedarwood – 4 drops

- Orange or Petgrain – 1 drop

- Palmarosa or Ylang Ylang – 1 drop

- Vetvier – 1 drop

This recipe is great for men as it smells like the woods and not too girly, women will love it too. Mix all the ingredients together in a diffuser and enjoy as your room fills with relaxing, stress relieving smells.

CHAPTER 3: AROMATHERAPY FOR BEAUTY

In a never ending quest for beauty, people have been drawn to potions, elixirs and magical tonics in hopes of attaining their ideal look. This, while sometimes leading to new discoveries, generally is not all it's cracked up to be. This is one of those exceptions. Aromatherapy can be used to improve your appearance quite significantly, but you must remember that this is not an overnight 'magic' quick fix, and must be used for some time, usually for a few weeks. Despite the downside of not working straight away, aromatherapy can refresh us, give us and our body's energy and make us feel and look our best.

Skin Issues

There are a multitude of various common skin issues we encounter in our everyday life that keep us annoyed and often make us have a poor body image. A common example is what you may have been struggling with – acne. With aromatherapy and it's consequent release of natural mixtures into your pores, cleaning them and not only lessening acne, but also preventing further breakouts, reformation of old acne as well as preventing acne scars. This is achievable through a range of simple, and easy to do at home recipes. These recipes will allow you to take good care of your skin, or reduce acne/rash at the comfort of your own house, and without expensive medication.

Another similar example of a skin condition that can be solved using either expensive treatments or aromatherapy is the seemingly inevitable formation of wrinkles. Aromatherapy releases natural oils under your skin through the pores which encourages blood flow, and thus regenerates your skin cells. These oils are also full of nutrients and proteins like collagen which helps the skin to maintain its firmness. This results in your skin looking healthy and rejuvenated after just a few days of usage.

When preparing a certain recipe, there is a simple rule to it – buy the oils that you are going to be using only from trusted suppliers, as the oils are the active ingredient, and so are extremely important for the recipes. Furthermore, remember that the oils have to be 100% pure, as additions of other chemicals may ruin the effect that the oils are intended to have. As a safety precaution remember to never put 100% pure oil directly on skin without first diluting the oil. This is very important, simply because all oils are very powerful by themselves and can thus burn your skin, or irritate it if used without dilution. It is also a good idea to test your solution on a small patch of unaffected area of your skin – commonly your wrist, as this procedure tests for potential irritation and/or allergies that you may not be aware of. In order for you to test for potential irritations, simply apply a little bit (often around 5 drops) of your mixture onto a cotton wad (which is easily available in any supermarket) and gently swipe your cotton wad over the area where you have decided to test, then wait 24 hours. If no irritation or rash occurred in that time, it is safe for you to use your mixture, and if any irritation or rash starts occurring, stop treatment immediately, as it can leave permanent marking on your skin, as well as damage the skin.

For the vast majority of these recipes, I recommend you getting a small plastic bottle to preserve the mixture that you prepared. These bottles are very easy to acquire, as they are simply sold in any drugstore in the traveling section. Storing most of these mixtures is very simple, as all you have to do is place them in your plastic bottle and keep them in a cool place, without high-intensity light, which is generally just any cupboard Before you use any of these mixtures, remember to follow a few simple steps:

Firstly, make sure you shake the mixture thoroughly, as the ingredients inside it may separate, and as they have to arrive and act together, this is a necessary step to insure the mixture working.

Secondly, clean your skin with warm water before applying the mixture, as dirt and dead skin can block pores, which will stop the oils from arriving to their destination. This will result in a severely decreased effect, if any at all.

Finally, take your time about these procedures – if you rush through them, there is a solid chance that you will misapply, or apply not enough of the mixture onto the affected area. If you take it slow, you will find that it doesn't take much time, and the effect is a lot better.

Most of these recipes ask you to use cotton balls or swabs, but a similar object is fine – like tissues, Q-tips or the like. The most important thing is for you to not, under any circumstances, use your hands as that can spread harmful bacteria across your skin, as well as introduce dirt.

Most of these mixtures should start working within the first 2-3 weeks, but if you don't see any improvement past that point feel free to go for a different version of the treatment. For instance, both Myrrh and Patchouli essential oils are beneficial to aging skin due to their proteins, so if the recipe only includes one and not the other, and isn't working, you should switch to the other, and try again. Remember, our bodies are different, and so each one will need an individual approach, so you should feel free to change the recipes up to suit your needs. As long as you do not apply undiluted oil, and there is no rash, burns or general discomfort, you should feel free to adjust any recipes given in this book to suit your needs. And remember, there should be no pain or discomfort when applying any of the mixtures!

Acne

Various oil used aromatherapy have both anti-bacterial and anti-inflammatory properties due to their unique structure and proteins, which helps you to treat acne, and acne related problems with them. It is incredibly important to never apply undiluted oils onto your skin, as essential oils are very, very powerful and will irritate your skin, or even give you a burn. Due to this, oftentimes 'less is more' in this case, as little positive impact is much better than severe negative impact which can happen if you make the oils too concentrated.

The recipe below can be used both as conventional oil (for rubbing in with a cotton ball) as well as a gel. If you prefer a gel, simply remove the Rose Hip oil and replace it with the same amount of Aloe Vera, which available at most drug stores. Aloe Vera in itself has anti-bacterial properties and can help reduce acne, but in combination with other oil can help to soothe the skin, and relieve the redness and swelling that you can experience from acne, or a similar skin condition.

Acne Abolisher Blend:

- Rose Hip oil – 5 tbsp
- Tea Tree oil – 7 drops
- Lemon oil – 7 drops
- Lavender oil – 5 drops
- Cedar oil – 2 drops

Simply add all the ingredients into the plastic bottles that you can buy from the drug store, and shake vigorously for 20 seconds, so that all the ingredients are mixed thoroughly. This mixing is required to insure equal spread of oil within the mixture. Before using this mixture, it is highly recommended that you clean your face with warm water, to remove any dirt and dead skin, and dry it. Then, take a cotton ball and wet it with clean, preferably pure, water and apply only a few drops of the mixture onto it via a pipette or a similar dripper. Remember: DO NOT apply pure oil to the affected area, as this will create irritation! After applying the mixture onto a cotton ball, slowly and steadily rub it in over the affected area. Do not apply a lot of pressure, rather, apply it slowly. Repeat the application twice a day. I generally prefer to do it in the morning and before I go to sleep, but the time of day is not very important for this particular mixture. This recipe will not only remove excessive moisture and sweat from the affected area; it will also use its antibacterial properties to relieve your skin of acne swelling and redness that is caused by bacteria. The Aloe Vera will also soothe your skin.

This mixture should be stored in a cool, dry and dark place. It can be kept for up to 6 month, as long as before applying it you will shake the bottle to re-mix all the contents.

*Please also note not to apply massage oil undiluted onto bare skin.

Age Spots

As we get older, many negative changes happen with our skin. Wrinkles start forming, and sun spots start appearing. They usually tend to appear as grey or brown spots where there is the most sun exposure, so generally on the arms, face, chest, back or legs. While not really dangerous in on themselves, sometimes they serve as warning sign for melanoma (skin cancer), so if you get a rapid increase in age spots. Otherwise, the treatment bellow is a cheap and simple way to solve your problem of dark spots by harnessing the power of essential oils. As with other recipes, excessive use of oil is going to be very damaging to your skin, so you will have to use a cotton ball for application on skin. This particular oil does not target, or is influenced by bacteria, so it can also be applied as a lotion by hand, after mixing with water in a bowl. If you don't mix it, this will damage your skin significantly! The most important aspect of this particular recipe is that you apply this lotion or oil to clean skin; otherwise its effects will be next to none.

Diminish Age Spots:

- Almond oil – 15 ml

- Argan oil - 15 ml

- Wheat Germ oil - 1 capsule

- Evening Primrose oil - 2 capsules

- Lavender oil - 10 drops

- Rose oil - 2 drops

This is another simple and straightforward recipe – simply mix the ingredients in a pre-purchased plastic bottle and shake well. The shaking is especially important in this recipe, as some of the oils will have different densities, and thus will not mix that easily compared to other ones. Unless you shake this mixture up really well, you are not going to achieve the best result.

1. Now, the way I usually do it, is to take a shower and thoroughly clean the areas where this mixture is going to be applied to and dry myself thoroughly.

2. After that, I either mix a few drops into a small bowl, or I take a cotton ball, wet in warm water and gently rub it in to affected areas.

It is recommended to repeat this procedure twice a day for optimal results, so you can take a shower in the morning, and simply wash your face and hands with warm water and apply the oil via a cotton ball during the evening. This will allow your age spots to dissipate, as these oils will change the concentration of melanin producing bodies, thus normalizing skin colour over a few weeks. After preparation and application, simply store this in a plastic bottle in a cupboard.

Age Spot Fader:

- Francinsense – 1 drop

- Carrot Seed – 1 drop

- Rosehip Oil – 1 tsp

Mix all of the oils into a small bowl and use a cotton bud or q-tip to apply the blend onto the affected areas. Do this twice a day until you start to see improvements.

Anti – Aging Serum:

- Rosehip Seed – 20 drops

- Carrot Seed – 20 drops

- Apricot Kernel Oil – 1 cup

Mix all ingredients and store in an amber bottle. Massage this serum onto a cleansed full face and neck and you can keep reusing this blend until you see results. Do this twice a week.

Cellulite

Cellulite is a bane of a lot of people, as it deforms the skin, leaving a terrible looking skin fool of bumps. Cellulite is basically just fat tissue pushing its way into other tissues, such as muscle and skin. Although there are some methods that make cellulite less visible, such as drinking lots of water, these just mask the problem. Other methods include keeping fit, which ultimately results in a decrease in fat tissue and thus in cellulite. But you must remember that these treatments are not exclusionary, and so have a much better effect when combined with the use of essential oils. The essential oils allow deep heat to enter the fat tissue, and thus assist breakdown of fat. The most important part of the recipe below is to take the time to massage it into the skin for several minutes once applied. This will allow deeper and more equal penetration and thus will help your body to take care of the fat tissue.

Detoxify for Cellulite:

- Rosemary – 10 drops
- Geranium – 10 drops
- Juniper – 20 drops
- Spearmint – 10 drops
- Grapefruit – 10 drops
- Grapeseed oil – 100ml

Mix this remedy into a bowl and massage onto your cellulite to stimulate circulation.

Cellulite Remover:

- Grapefruit oil - 20 drops
- Juniper Berry oil - 20 drops
- Rosemary Oil - 20 drops
- Sweet almond oil – 6 tbsp

The instructions on how to use this oil mixture is very similar to the previous ones described as all you have to do to prepare it is simply to mix it in a bottle that you should have bought from an average drug store in the travel section.

1. For this mixture, it is more important than ever to clean your skin thoroughly, and shake the bottle before using, as the oils have to go down through the pores the longest compared to all of the other mixtures.

2. After cleaning your skin thoroughly, simply apply a small amount onto a pad, or a cotton ball. After this, remember to rub this mixture into the affected area for approximately 10-15 minutes, twice a day.

This mixture acts very simply, as oils enter the pores; they drop off key proteins into deposits of fat, and thus help the organism to naturally break apart. Thus, this simple solution proposed by aromatherapy, helps your body to deal with the cellulite by itself, not via a surgical operation or other chemicals. Remember to never apply pure oil to affected areas, as you are running the risk of having a chemical burn, which will scour the skin, at the same time making pores smaller, and thus making further treatment impossible and dangerous. If you have any signs of irritation, immediately stop and either dilute the mixture more, or contact a professional.

Chapped Lips

We are all aware of the annoying feeling we get when our lips dry up and crack. Our skin on the lips is incredibly thin, and with blood vessels being incredibly close to the surface, chapped lips can be a pain, literally. When our lips get dried up, we tend to lick them. This, surprisingly, only exacerbates the problem, as saliva is slightly acidic, and thus destroys the ultra-thin skin that covers our lips.

Here are a few reasons why chapped lips are better off being treated with an aromatherapy-esque cure:

- Most lip balms and/or chapsticks tend to only surround the lips with a moistening effects, while this aromatherapy based treatment actually helps the body to repair the skin

- This treatment does not have a bad taste that most of the chapsticks and the like have

- This treatment is cheap, and easy to make at home

Overall, this balm provides a fast and effective solution to chapped lips compared to many conventional chapsticks and lip balms.

Lip Hydrator:

- Orange – 10 drops
- Beeswax – 3 tsp
- Coconut Oil – 4.5 tsp
- Shea Butter – 1.5 tsp
- Jojoba Oil – 1.5 tsp

This recipe should make 12, 5ml lip balms. You can buy 5 ml DIY lip balm tubes on eBay or your local arts and crafts store and add the mixture into those and store in the fridge until they have hardened.

Deep Lip Therapy:

- Jojoba oil – 10ml
- Castor oil – 5ml
- Argan oil - 5ml
- Wheat germ oil - 2 capsules
- 50ml bottle – pre bought from any pharmacy.

The preparation for this mixture and its application is slightly different from the others described above. The key difference lies in the application process – compared to other mixtures outlined above, this mixture has to be applied by a Q-tip, or a similar device, which was soaked in warm water and had a drop of the mixture applied to it.

1. But first, to prepare this mixture, which is quite simple – just get a plastic 50 ml bottle, fill it with these oils and shake it for a few minute. Shaking is not as important, as the oils should mix easily.

2. After preparation, simply apply a drop of the mixture onto a Q-tip that has been soaked in warm water, and apply it to dry areas of the lips. After this, simply re–apply this every time you have been outside for an extended period of time to ensure rapid healing of the tissue.

Just remember, that despite the taste not being bad, it is not very healthy to eat a lot of this mixture, as castor oil has a laxative effect. After using this mixture, simply store it in a cool, dry place like a cupboard. This storing method will ensure preservation of key proteins that make this process possible. Before using it, remember to shake the bottle well, just in case the mixture has separated, especially if you haven't used it in a few months' time. This will ensure a uniform delivery across your lips, giving you the best and fastest recovery from dried lips.

Dandruff

A lot of us have been, or are, being bothered by dandruff – that white small stuff that keeps appearing on our hair, and we can't get rid of it. We all have tried various solutions to this problem, from various advertised "anti-dandruff" shampoos to getting a different haircut. It seems that none of these products are effective. This solution to dandruff, on the other hand, is very reliable, tested by time and people. This cure based on aromatherapy, as well as healing effects of essential oils, penetrates your skin, and solves the problem of dandruff (which is the skin peeling off) by rejuvenating the skin of your scalp. This treatment soothes your skin too due to Lavender oil and has an anti-inflammatory and anti-bacterial effect, due to the nature of the tea tree oil. This allows supreme cleansing of your scalp, which would otherwise be impossible. What is the best part is that this treatment is available to you for a low price, as you can easily make it yourself!

Dandruff Defiance:

- Coconut Oil – 30 drops

- Lavender Essential Oil – 5 drops

- Lemon Essential Oil - 8 drops

- Tea Tree Essential Oil – 4 drops

1. The preparation of this mixture is very similar to the one used against acne - just mix the oils in a 50ml bottle that is available from any pharmacy, thus insuring the same thickness across the entire liquid, which means that it will spread out a lot better and more evenly compared to not mixed one.

2. To use this cure, all you have to do is after using your normal shampoo, apply to your hair as you would conditioner, making sure to massage it into your scalp as best as possible.

3. Let it sit in five minutes while you go about your normal shower routine. After five minutes, wash out thoroughly.

Remember to never apply the oil undiluted, as they will burn the sensitive skin of your scalp, which can lead to a huge range of problems. Be sure to was the mixture out thoroughly, otherwise you are risking irritation. This solution basically is aimed to activate your cells reproductive mechanism, rejuvenating them, by throwing down the right proteins through the pores, as well as increasing the blood flow, thus allowing easy movement of materials. You have to store this mixture in a dark and dry place, like a cupboard, as well as remember to shake the bottle before using. This will allow a better delivery of nutrients.

Dry skin

Dry skin is a very common skin condition, generally caused by either excessive use of soap (especially on areas with thin skin, like face) or excessive heat/sun exposure. Dry skin is relatively easy to deal with, as it readily absorbs any and all oils applied to it. On the down side, it is much more sensitive compared to oily skin, and will hurt a lot if any irritation was to happen. This mixture aims to allow your sebaceous glands (the ones that moisturize your skin) to activate and start working, instead of artificially creating moisture that will not last long, and does not prompt your body to take any action, instead doing the opposite. This mixture allows a free passage if nutrients into the sebaceous glands as well as the skin cells, thus allowing them to experience the change from being dry to moisturized smoothly without any side effects. The recipe for this mixture is very simple, just take

Dry Skin Scrub

- Peppermint – 2 drops

- Lavender – 6 drops

- Oatmeal – 2 tbsp

- Cornmeal – 1 tbsp

Grind all of the dry ingredients in a blender. Then add in the essential oils and mix well. Pour into a container and store in the fridge. When you're ready to use, apply onto wet skin (where affected).

Dry Skin Relieving Moisturizer:

- Coconut oil – 30 drops

- Roman Chamomile essential oil - 25 drops

- Jasmine - 6 drops

- Geranium - 6 drops

1. Blend these oils together in a pre-purchased bottle, until the oils are indistinguishable from one another.

2. This is incredibly simple to do - just shake the bottle well for a few minutes, and as the oils are similar, they will intermix.

3. After this, simply clean the area which is dry, but do not use soap, simply use hot water, as the soap will dry the skin out even more. After that, simply take a pad or a cotton wad, dip it into warm clean water, and apply a droplet of the mixture onto it.

This is one of the cases where you have to be extremely carefully, as dry skin will burn easily, even if the oils are diluted. Make sure that you rub the oils in carefully, and wash your face if it starts being itchy or burning. For optimal effect, perform this procedure twice a day, and rub the oils in slowly, so that they diffuse well. Remember that dry skin is an effect of a different problem, and while aromatherapy will allow you to recover quickly, you may need to consider changing your habits, as ultimately they lead to skin drying out. Here are a few tips:

• Keep your face protected from strong winds or heat, as they can dry out your skin so quick that you will not even notice it until it's too late

• Wear sunscreen, as the sun and UV radiation can dry skin out too

• Avoid washing your face with body wash, as the skin on your face is gentle and will be burnt by the chemicals that are meant to clean our thicker skins on backs/hands.

Nails

Everyone wants to have strong, beautiful and we'll looking nails, but often times people think that their nails cannot be improved. This can be no further from the truth, as this simple recipe will fix your nails, and make them more shiny and more healthy looking. This recipe will easily do this, as it will help your body to release keratin, which is a main part of nails. After that, the keratin can easily help your fingernails take the right shape, as well as to stop discoloration of the nails. The lemon grass essential oil will also soothe your skin around nails, thus making your fingers look great. This is especially useful if you play an instrument where a lot of attention is going to be placed onto fingers - like the piano, guitar or the like. By healing the bad-looking skin you will not only boost your general looks, but also remove the risk of diseases, as the wounds or irritations through with bacteria could enter are no longer present on your hands. This means that this is a great thing to do, not only because of beauty, but also because of health reasons. With this Simple, easy to make at home mixture, you will achieve the nails that you wanted in just a few weeks time! The recipe is very simple, simply take

Nail Moisturizer:

- Lavender – 4 drops

- Bay Leaf – 2 drops

- Sandalwood - 3 drops

- Jojoba oil – 3 tsp

Soak nails in this blend for 10 minutes to regain moisture in the nails. Then buff to stimulate circulation and bring out a healthy shine.

Nail Nourisher:

- Lemon essential oil – 2 drops

- Water – 1 cup

1. Pour the cup of water into a bowl, enough that you will be able to place your fingers into it. Use warm water, as this will lead to the best absorption by skin.

2. After placing 2 drops into the bowl, place your fingers into the bowl. After soaking, put additional 2 drops of lemon oil over soaked nails and massage it in slowly, making sure to massage the cuticle all the way up to the nail tip.

This will ensure that the cells will absorb the oil, and thus will rejuvenate these cells, and thus allow them to produce keratin, which will allow your nails to look good. Once done, complete the process over again for your other hand. This process will heal your cells, and help your nail to accept the way that you want them to grow, as when you will cut them, they will not shatter due to the unique proteins in the lemon essential oil. This further strengthens your nails, and makes them the right color. Be aware that the nails should be soaked in water for a while (at least ten minutes) to get the best results. As this is reusable, simply store the lemon essential oil in a plastic bottle, and add it when you want to use it. it is recommended that you repeat this procedure every day, two times a day.

Oily Hair

We all have struggled with oily hair - that disgusting feeling of your hair just sticking to stuff, and none of the shampoos helping. Oily Hair is quite a common problem, that has the same root cause as oily and dry skin. As the sebaceous glands start producing too much sebum (oil), the hair and the skin can't deal with it, often making the skin and hair oily and sticky. Ironically, this problem can be solved using oils and a little bit of aromatherapy. The ylang ylang oil will allow better drainage of sebum, while lemon grass oil will soothe your skin and make your sebaceous glands more relaxed. Jojoba oil will simply act as a calming presence for your skin, as it will make your cells that produce sebum work slower. This will ultimately lead to dissipation of excessive sebum, and thus hair becoming normal again, only after a week or two. The recipe for this mixture is quite simple, but the preparation is slightly different to the rest.

Oily Hair Control:

- Jojoba oil – 20 ml

- Lemon Grass Oil – 1 drop

- Ylang Ylang Oil – 2 drops

1. First, take the oil and mix them together thoroughly. They should be if the sand thickness when you are done. This is needed to insure equal spread over your scalp.

2. After this, all you have to do is after using your normal shampoo, simply tub this mixture into your scalp, much like with the mixture against the dandruff.

3. Let this mixture stay into your hair for a few minutes, while you clean up. After five minutes, wash out thoroughly.

Definitely, do not, ever apply this oil by itself without shampoo, and/or without water. This will irritate and possibly burn the sensitive scalp, which can create a huge amounts of problems, such as formation of acne (as pores will be blocked). After applying the shampoo mixed with the oil mixture, you should note improvement in a few weeks time, but stop if yours skin gets irritated, as it will cause a lot of problems, which will be difficult to solve.

Wrinkles

Wrinkles seem to be an unavoidable onslaught of old age - with older skin not being able to support itself, it limps and thus creates wrinkles. It seems that nothing, bar the most expensive surgeries can stop this slow and steady advancement of old age, with people getting, and looking older. Wrinkles became a sort of a definition of someone's age. Then, you probably will find it interesting that the wrinkling is reversible, using aromatherapy. The idea lies in delivering essential oils which contain structures akin to collagen and thus, but preparing this simple, quick and overall versatile treatment, one can completely reverse any and all signs of ageing. This is because the essential oils simply go through your pores and drop off these structures, allowing your cells to regenerate, and give your skin that young and healthy look. While this sounds incredibly complex in theory, it is actually very simple, as all that you have to do is to get

Anti-Aging Wrinkle Remover:

- Olive oil – 3 tbsp
- Geranium oil – 2 drops
- Lavender oil – 3 drops
- Carrot oil - 3 drops
- Fennel Oil – 1 drop

Because of the large number of various compounds within this mixture it is more importantly than ever before to shake it thoroughly, as well as shake it any time that you are going to use it. This is required to ensure the delivery of collagen like structures into the pores.

1. After preparing the mixture, and mixing it thoroughly, all you have to do is get a bowl of warm water and clean your face, or wherever you are going to be applying this mixture to.

2. Then, dip your q-tip, cotton ball or a pad (depends on the area where you are going to be applying the mixture too, for small areas it's recommended to use a q-tip, while a cotton ball works for larger ones) and slowly rub the mixture diluted with water in.

Remember that you must not apply the oils without diluting them and in this particular case, less is often more - simply because if you apply too much oil, your skin will not handle it and will most likely become oily and sticky, while not getting rid of the wrinkles. The best way to take care of your skin with this to simply use a little bit at a time, twice a day. This will ensure a smooth transition for your skin, and reduce the chance of it becoming oily.

Overall, aromatherapy has a multitude of applications, whether it is to make you more beautiful or not. For this particular branch, the importantly thing to remember is that nothing should hurt, and if it does, then you are something wrong. To get the best results, all you have to do is buy quality oils, follow the instructions for the first few times and then, when you get used to aromatherapy, adjust the recipes so that they work best for you, as all of us are different, and we have different needs.

CHAPTER 4: AROMATHERAPY FOR HOME

The practicality of aromatherapy is wide ranging and the everyday household uses of aromatherapy are often overlooked, from mood elevation to cleaning products. Though what is truly phenomenal is the ease in which you can create your own personalized, all natural therapeutic remedies at home.

The following chapter will outline a number of different uses for aromatherapy around the home, with a focus on both its practical and therapeutic nature, while also explaining the most beneficial methods of application. The more tried, true and popular options will be discussed as examples of the benefits of using aromatherapy in the everyday life. The sphere of aromatherapy is wide ranging and there are many more options than are discussed here in this chapter.

Some of the many benefits of conventional aromatherapy are that it can change the entire mood of a room, help you begin your day with vigour and then assist you in getting a restful sleep. The brilliance of aromatherapy is in its versatility and variety, there is a remedy for any situation to suit any taste. Subsequently, the necessity for aromatherapy is certainly not uniform to one type across a home, hence why we are providing you with an array of ideas to suit most any mood or situation.

Applicator Varieties

The methods of use vary depending on the desired result. The oil burner, scented wax and potpourri varieties are popular methods for achieving a lasting aroma. The benefit of these types of application are that they create wide spread aerial diffusion.

The use of scented oil and wax is generally used with the aid of a potpourri bowl suspended above a candle, this is to melt the wax or heat the oil and release the aroma. The obstacle generally with these kinds of applicators is the ratio and amounts of ingredient being used, too much will create an overwhelming scent, too little will be a waste. Although this is again a matter of personal preference, there are general guidelines that should ensure the aroma created is pleasant and enjoyable.

The use of aroma remedies also allows for the creation and use of homemade air freshening sprays, there is limited expertise required for this and it should be again made to preference. All that is required is a small clean spray bottle (size 150 mL) with ¼ cup of distilled water mixed with ¼ of high proof alcohol (vodka works well), and finally the addition of 35 – 40 drops of scented oil(s). Gently mix and allow it to sit for a short period of time, until the ingredients are settled and cured.

Using reed diffusers is easy in that all that is required is to put the reed sticks into the scented oil. Once one end of the reed has been dipped and saturated in oil, flip the saturated side up and have it in the air, allowing the dry side to be saturated for when it is time to flip the reed sticks over again. In essence by doing this, the saturated ends of the reed sticks are in open air and in turn release a soft fragrance across the room. When the saturation has dried, flip the sticks back over and expose the freshly saturated side to the air. This should be done as necessary, though every 2 - 3 days is effective. It should also be noted that the more reed sticks being used the stronger the scent will be, though a maximum of 12 and minimum of 4 is a good rule of thumb.

For the use of scented oils between, drop 2 - 7 drops into the diffuser bowl depending on the strength of aroma desired. Furthermore, 1 - 3 drops of your favourite essential oil may also be added onto a fragrant candle or scented wax for additional qualities. To do this, the candle should be left to burn for 5 – 10 minutes and then extinguished before adding 1 – 2 drops of oil onto the melted wax before reigniting. This achieves a lasting scent, and is especially pleasurable when added to an already scented candle. The aroma created by this method is also quite strong, hence its use should generally be in the kitchen, living room or any area with open space that will allow the scent to disperse and settle evenly.

Air Freshening

It's not a secret that all odours are pleasant to the senses. Often we cover up unpleasant smells with sweet smelling sprays without thinking of the hazardous potential of spraying synthetic chemicals across the room.

Aromatherapy can provide is both a more natural and far more pleasant scent than these chemical sprays. You can make aromatherapy remedies to your preference in your own home as a more natural and beneficial option.

The versatility when creating an aromatherapy remedy is advantageous in itself as there are few limitations on what can be used in creating a pleasing mixture; from essential oils derived from flowers, herbs or wood can be used. You can mix the essential oils with water to make a room spray or drop them into a diffuser to fill the room with the scent. Try one of these recipes to freshen up the air in any room.

Spicy Chai Air Freshener

- Cardamom – 4 drops

- Cassia – 3 drops

- Clove – 3 drops

- Ginger – 2 drops

Mix all the oils together in a diffuser, or mix with ¼ cup of water and use in a spray bottle.

Summer Citrus Air Freshener

- Orange – 5 drops

- Lemon – 5 drops

- Lime – 5 drops

- Grapefruit – 5 drops

Mix all the oils together in a diffuser, or mix with ¼ cup of water and use in a spray bottle.

Living Areas and Bedrooms

The options of oil diffusion are not limited to the use of a diffuser bowl or candle; their versatility allows them to also be delivered through steam. To achieve this one should simply boil 1 – 2 cups of water and add between 4 -10 drops of scented oil depending on decided strength of odour. This process allows the essential oils added to bind with the steam already created by the boiled water, in turn generating an aromatic steam that can fill a room or area of the home.

This method creates a less powerful aroma than those influenced by flame, which in turn allows them to be useful in the smaller rooms of the house. A particularly good use of the steam diffusion method is to induce a relaxing aroma prior to going to sleep, or upon waking to generate vigour and wakefulness.

Living Room Calming Steam Blend

- Roman Chamomile – 4 drops

- Lavender – 3 drops

- Clary Sage – 2 drops

- Geranium – 2 drops

- Ylang Ylang – 1 drop

Drop the essential oils into a bowl full of 1 – 2 cups of freshly boiled water. Place in the centre of the room for the oils to disperse.

Another popular application of aromatherapy that is advised for bedrooms and living areas is the use of reed diffusers or reed sticks. The benefit of a reed diffuser is that it is something that can be left unchecked for a longer period of time than that of candles or steam diffusers. The advantage of using reed diffusers is that they are appropriate for any room in the house; they can create a relaxing atmosphere in the bedroom or living area.

A further use of essential oils can be the simple application of 1 – 3 drops onto a tissue or cloth to create a handy, portable aromatherapy applicator. This follows also to applying therapeutic oils to a pillow case for an enhanced night sleep or even the collar of a shirt or blouse for residual benefits across the day. The use of an aroma spray is particularly good for creating a welcoming aroma in the living areas of the home, or aiding in relaxation in the bedroom. It can be sprayed on furniture or directly onto your bed linens.

Pillow And Sheet Aromatherapy Spray

- Lavender – 4 drops
- Roman Chamomile – 4 drops
- Vetvier – 1 drop
- ¼ cup distilled water
- spray bottle

Using a small spray bottle, drop the essential oils into the water and gently shake. Spray once onto your pillows and a few times on your bed linens.

Bathroom and Bathing

You can create a relaxing and soothing bathing experience with the addition of essential oils to your bath water. Prior to adding the essential oils to a bath, they should be mixed with a carrier oil to allow the essential oils to dissolve into the water, rather than settling and sitting at the top. Carrier oils are also a great addition to help moisturize your skin. Soak in the bath for 20 – 30 minutes, but no longer as there can be minor irritation if one's skin is exposed for prolonged periods to some types of oils.

Relaxing Aromatherapy Bath Oil Recipe

- Sandalwood – 30 drops
- Lavender – 12 drops
- Cedarwood – 2 drops
- Carrier Oil – 4 oz

Combine all the oils into a dark glass jar. Shake gently before your bath. Use about one tablespoon for each bath. The mixture will store up to 3 months.

There is also an advantage to using reed diffusers in the bathroom as they can create a relaxing atmosphere when bathing, while also being just as good at covering bathroom odours with a fresh though subtle aroma.

Spray aromas are again very useful as an air freshener in the bathroom, as the aerial dispersion is an easy cover for bathroom odours, leaving the bathroom smelling and feeling fresh and clean.

Deodorizing Air Freshener

- Lemon – 8 drops

- Eucalyptus – 6 drops

- Tea Tree – 4 drops

Mix all the oils together in a diffuser, or mix with ¼ cup of water and use in a spray bottle.

Moreover, as the scent generated by candle based applicators is strong and lasting, the benefits are of good use in the bathroom to not only cover bathroom odours, but to also create a calming environment when bathing to unwind and relax.

Kitchen

The use of aromatherapy spray in the kitchen is easy to make and can help cover up smells from fatty foods and cleaning products. Spraying and aromatherapy spray in the kitchen can help keep the food smells from lingering on your clothes. No one likes the smell of fried onions and garlic sticking to them after they've left the kitchen.

Kitchen Odour Replacing Spray

- Rosemary – 2 drops
- Eucalyptus – 2 drops
- Lime – 2 drops
- Lavender – 2 drops
- ¼ cup distilled water
- ¼ cup vodka
- spray bottle

Use a small, clean spray bottle to gently mix all the ingredients together. Spray around the kitchen as needed.

Many essential oils have powerful anti-fungal and anti-bacterial properties. Essential oils are much safer than store bought chemical cleaners because they are natural and plant-derived. Citrus based oils are most notable for the fact that they are anti-septic and anti-bacterial in nature, making it great to use in bathrooms and kitchens.

Add in 10 drops of a citrus oil, like grapefruit, lemon or orange, to your dish soap to make doing the dishes more enjoyable. You'll rest well knowing the dishes were extra clean with the anti-bacterial essential oils.

To wipe down the counters, cupboards and the stove top, try dropping 8 drops of essential oil directly to your dish cloth to really clean the surfaces. The best essential oils for the job are: thyme, pine, lavender, lemon and eucalyptus.

Reed sticks are again recommended as their long period of usage allows for a fresh scent to be always present in the kitchen, and in turn allows for the odour of food stuffs to be combated with ease and limited repeat application.

Although the use of aromatherapy in the kitchen is again very much up to the individual and the reason for use, there are times when a diffuser bowl or wax burner may be of necessity if the smell of food stuffs is strong, like especially odorous seafood. The use of oil or wax burners can also be useful in the kitchen as a tool for wakefulness, by igniting an aroma remedy like that of peppermint for instance, the invigorating properties of the aroma will assist in preparing a person for the day ahead.

Moods and Uses

The versatility of aromatherapy also provides an array of personal benefits; as different scents can evoke different moods for different scenarios, you can create an atmosphere to suit any demand. There is a wealth of great options when choosing the type a type of fragrance and at times this can be the most difficult part of devising your own aromatherapy remedies at home. To help ease the burden of choice, the tried and true scents are as follows.

Mood Elevation

To elevate your mood, you can chose citrus scented essential oils because they have anti-depressant characteristics. The scent is strong but not overwhelming and is attributed to uplifting both individual and atmospheric moods.

A further aid in combating anxiety and mood issues is the use of rose in aromatherapy. The strong sweet aroma the intoxicating scent of rose oil is perfect for use at the end of a long day. Assisting in unwinding, the use of rose aromas are perfect for relaxing or sensual bathing, and can assist in the relief of insomnia if placed in the bedroom.

Application methods range in use from petals or oils and their compatibility with any diffuser option, or alternatively the use of droplets onto a tissue placed in your pillow can allow for prolonged benefits. The scent of rose can be quite strong though rarely overpowering, it is recommended to begin usage at a lower dose until preferred aroma is found.

A great base aroma for living areas or bedrooms is the ylang ylang flower, it's enticing scent is subtle though calming. Best used in small doses ylang ylang has been said to cause minor headaches in some users if the concentration of oils/ dry herb is too high. Recommended application is through steam diffusion as it allows the scent to spread without centralizing, and allows for well-rounded aerial diffusion.

The use of ylang ylang is also prominently applied through the use of reed sticks, as the slow and consistent release of aroma when using reed diffusers is perfect when couple with the nature of the ylang ylang scent.

The benefit of the ylang ylang essential oil is in its calming properties. Recommended during periods of stress, ylang ylang is a great addition to any mood elevating mix, and is itself attributed to aid in anger management.

Mood Elevating Aromatherapy Mix:

- Bergamot – 3 drops
- Ylang Ylang – 1 drop
- Grapefruit – 1 drop

Drop the essential oils into a diffuser, or dip reed sticks into the oils, and place in a room to improve your mood.

Aromatherapy For Happiness Mix:

- Sandalwood – 2 drops
- Bergamot – 2 drops
- Rose – 1 drop

Drop the essential oils into a diffuser, or dip reed sticks into the oils, and place in a room to feel happier.

Vigour and Wakefulness

When using peppermint in aromatherapy is best applied through steam diffusing methods or via a freshener spray, as the aroma can be quite strong. However if one's preference is to prolong and maintain the robust aroma, the suggested method of application is the use of a diffusion bowl and candle.

The subsequent benefits of using peppermint aroma remedies are again ranging and varied. Peppermint is especially good to use in the morning because it helps you wake up as the scent is invigorating. Peppermint promotes mental stamina and clarity, while also being thought to assist in alleviating fatigue. It should be carefully noted that while peppermint aroma remedies can assist in mental alertness they at the same time have the ability to therefore hinder restfulness if used too close to sleep. A final attribute of peppermint aroma is that it can act as an aphrodisiac.

The use of rosemary in aromatherapy is another reliable staple. Rosemary can be used in oils or dry herb applicators. Rosemary can be used through steam diffusing, reed sticks and droplets onto a tissue or diffuser candle. However reed sticks are further recommended as they allow the scent to maintain subtlety throughout the day without getting overly potent.

When using rosemary oil either as an inhalant or on a candle it should be noted that the aroma of rosemary is quite strong and lasting meaning a conservative approach to application is recommended until preferred strength of aroma is known.

The benefits of rosemary are varied, though when used aromatically the most noted benefits are that of increased concentration, mental clarity and focus. Subsequently you can also use rosemary in the mornings to assist in waking. Moreover the application of rosemary scented oils to a tissue or shirt collar on long car drives can assist in focus and wakefulness, this also applies when reading, studying or working to aid in the maintenance of cognitive focus across prolonged periods.

Rosemary can moreover be used as in a mood elevating aroma blend as its invigorating qualities can assist in sensory stimulation and subsequent mental vigour.

Invigorating Aromatherapy Blend:

- Peppermint – 2 drops

- Lemon – 2 drops

- Frankincense – 1 drop

Drop the essential oils into a diffuser, or dip reed sticks into the oils, and place in a room to feel invigorated.

Awaken Aromatherapy Blend:

- Rosemary – 2 drops

- Orange – 2 drops

Drop the essential oils into a diffuser, dip reed sticks into the oils, or place onto a tissue to inhale. As the oils are dispersed you will start to feel awakened.

Relaxation

Lavender is arguably the most used ingredient in mainstream aromatherapy and for good reason because it has an amazing aroma that can be used anywhere in home. It can cover bathroom or kitchen smells, create a warm and crisp atmosphere in living areas and can also aid in relaxation and sleep. The application of lavender oils ranges from steam diffusion, the use of reed sticks, diffusion candles, inhaling or soaking in baths.

The aroma of lavender is of medium strength which makes it a good base scent when creating relaxation mixes, though is efficient on its own. Applying a drop of lavender oil to a tissue and placing the tissue in your pillowcase is recommended to help you relax after a long and tiring day.

Do be careful though, lavender is generally a relaxing aroma, however if you use it in higher doses it can generate a more stimulating affect. Due to its rich scent lavenders versatility becomes evident in the fact that it can also be used in an air freshening spray to cover bathroom, kitchen or general odours.

Sandalwood is a great scent to relax and unwind with. It is recommended to be used through steam diffusing to allow the scent of spread across a room, though it is an aroma that can be applied through any method. The therapeutic benefits of using sandalwood are found in its subtle aroma that is attributed to enhanced moods and an aid when distressed or anxious. The calming and cleansing properties of sandalwood can also act as an aphrodisiac, and is recommended also for use in the bedroom or bath for sensual purposes, as well as simple relaxation purposes.

While many aroma remedies are attributed to aid in relaxation, it is chamomile that is the centrepiece of calming properties. You can use chamomile during times of stress, irritability and frustration. Chamomile is incredibly versatile in application methods, as it can found in anything from tea to scented waxes and oils.

The preferred method of use as the scent of chamomile is a medium to strong odour is through reed diffusers as their continuous, slow release of scent is optimal. The use of steam or diffusers is also recommended though only if the preferred aroma is that of a stronger and more abrasive scent.

Chamomile is also fantastic in aiding insomnia, so the use of reed sticks, or dry herb diffusers in the bedroom is a recommended application, as is oil droplets onto a tissue inside your pillowcase prior to sleep. To aid in the relieving of stress, chamomile can also be used when bathing, or meditating, as it truly is a very versatile and useful tool in aromatherapy and should be a staple ingredient in any relaxation mixture. It follows that the use of chamomile fragrances can also aid in child rearing, if a child is irritable and restless the application of chamomile to the room of the child can assist in calming and inducing sleep.

It must be said that there are many more ingredients in aromatherapy and that the most popular scents and methods of application have been discussed above in an effort to inspire you to create and personalize your home for different situations.

Aromatherapy itself is a forever-expanding domain as it is no longer just sweet smelling oils, as it can be personally stylized to fit the individual. It should also be noted that the use of many aroma remedies have multiple benefits and there is subsequently an immense amount of crossover in usage.

Calming Massage Oil:

- Chamomile – 8 drops

- Lavender – 5 drops

- Bergamot – 4 drops

- Clary Sage – 2 drops

Mix together all the oils in dark glass jar, dropping onto a tissue to inhale and feel relaxed. Alternatively you can mix with 2 ounces of a carrier oil to use in the bath or as a massage oil.

General Purpose Cleaning, Laundry, Glass and Window Cleaner

The use of aromatherapy when cleaning is very much overlooked in the field of aromatherapy in general. Not only are the aroma remedies all natural but they are versatile and reliable when cleaning. From general purpose cleaning to laundry to window cleaners, the use of aroma remedies can aid in creating a fresh smelling, germ free environment in the home.

General Purpose Cleaning

For general purpose cleaning the use of a spray bottle is generally the best applicator and the process is similar to that of creating a spray air freshener. All that is needed is a spray bottle, preferably unused or untainted with any sort of bleach or chemical product.

The method of creation is dependent on the size of the spray bottle though a generally good process is first to mix ¾ cup of white vinegar with 1 1/3 cup of warm – hot water. The next step is based on preference, whether you choose eucalyptus, citrus, pine or clove, add 7 – 10 drops of oil mixture and allow it to sit for a brief period.

If the odour is not strong enough, simply add more scented oil, though it is recommended to start with smaller amounts before working toward ones preferred amount. A similar process can be used in creating a sink or toilet disinfectant where 40 – 60 millilitres of preferred aroma oil should be added to around a litre of warm water.

Glass and Window Cleaning

To create a homemade aromatherapy window cleaner, a spray bottle is again recommended. Of course there is no limit on which essential oil can be added. Some of the best essential oils for cleaning are lemon, grapefruit, tea tree oil and lavender. It should be noted that if adding oil to cleaning products, do so sparingly as it can create a greasy overcoat if too much is added, do not add more than 5 drops as this is enough to create a pleasing aroma without ruining the mixture.

Glass Cleaning Mixture:

- 4 tablespoons vinegar
- 4 cups water
- 5 drops essential oil, lemon, lavender or tea tree oil

Mix all the ingredients together in a spray bottle. Spray onto glass and wipe with paper towel or a cloth.

Grout and Stain Scrub

Most aroma cleaning applications thus far have been spray based though there are ways of creating a scrub for hard to remove stains. Making the following recipe for an aromatherapy scrub will create a gritty paste perfect for removing burnt or dried food stuffs or even mould and mildew from your bathroom. This can be a mixture of scents or a single type, below are recommended oils but you can put almost any you like. By doing so, the scent is personalized to preference and leaves an enjoyably natural odour.

Aromatherapy Cleaning Scrub:

- 1 cups baking soda

- 2 tablespoons water

- Pea-size of liquid soap

- 6 drops essential oil, lemon, peppermint or tea tree oil

Mix the ingredients together to make a paste. Using a cloth put some paste on your stain and scrub. Rinse with water after.

Laundry

The versatility of aromatherapy is further evident in the fact it can also be a great natural supplement for laundry detergent. Though harder to make, the economical benefits are well worth the effort. Furthermore the rinse cycle can be aided by the addition of a half of a cup of tea tree oil or white vinegar and 2 – 3 drops of essential oil. This gives your clothes a lovely faint smell after being washed and in turn is also attributed to aiding in fabric softening. Washing with oils can leave a scent in fabrics, this is incredibly useful if when washing pillow cases, sheets and blankets a choice of oil like that of rose is added, as the residual aroma left in the fabrics will potentially reap prolonged benefits.

Aromatherapy Laundry Soap:

- 500 grams baking soda

- 2 tablespoons water

- 20 drops essential oil, can be equal parts orange and geranium or lavender and vanilla

Mix all the ingredients together to make a laundry paste that will dissolve when you put it in the washing machine. You can make any combination of essential oils that you would like your fabrics to smell like after they are washed.

Usage and Application

Like aromatherapy as an air freshener, the use of essential oils in cleaning can create a vibrant and welcoming mood in the home. Depending on preference, there are numerous essences that remove germs, clean and create lasting aromas in and around the home. By harnessing the prior explained applications when cleaning a home can leave a pleasant and resonating atmosphere with every clean.

Multi Purpose Use

The use of citrus is one of the more useful remedies when using aroma therapeutic properties in cleaning because of its numerous benefits. Citrus based cleaning products are useful in both the kitchen and bathrooms as it can effectively combat foodstuffs, mildew and mould because of its acidic properties.

Citrus based aromatics are best applied through a spray when cleaning glass or wiping down benches and sinks in the kitchen, though also useful as a scrub when cleaning grime from ovens, stoves, showers, baths and toilets. Regardless of method of application the use of citrus based cleaning aromatics will leave a fresh and lasting scent, while in no way jeopardising the desired cleanliness.

Floors and Surface Areas

The pungent essence of tea tree oil is enough to show the intense variety of beneficial properties of the plant. Used for hundreds of years, tea tree oil is renowned for its anti-septic and anti-bacterial properties, meaning it is a perfect addition to any cleaning spray or scrub. Especially when used in cleaning the bathroom as it not only lifts stains and combats mould and mildew, but also leaves a fresh scent that reflects the cleanliness of a room without leaving it smelling overly sterile or bleached.

Though due to tea tree oil's strong scent, you probably want to keep it away from where meals are prepared or served as the intensity of its odour can be residual and is not a nice addition to food if used in the kitchen. As tea tree is as previously mentioned naturally anti-bacterial, it is of especially good use during cold and flu season, as it not only kills germs but is also aromatic enough to assist in clearing ones sinuses.

Tea tree oil should always be stored in a cool, dark place because direct light can hinder its properties. Begin with small dosages of tea tree oil and work toward ones preferred amount. A notable side benefit of cleaning with tea tree is that it acts as a natural insect repellent, so the use of tea tree cleaning products on outdoor areas and windows may be recommended purely for that reason alone.

Benches and Cooking Areas

Another popular aromatic oil to assist in cleaning is the use of pine, and for good reason. Pine produces not only a fresh aroma, but is also highly anti-bacterial and a brilliant disinfectant. The versatility of pine is advantageous, as it can be used in cleaning sprays scrubs or aromatically through reed and steam diffusers, as well as air freshening sprays.

Though as a cleaning product the anti-bacterial properties of pine coupled with its low toxicity levels makes it a great ingredient in general aromatic cleaning product. Use in the kitchen is recommended as the properties of pine both kills germs and leaves a refreshing though not overwhelming scent of cleanliness.

Perfect for glass cleaning, due to pine being a naturally thinner oil there is lesser chance residual marks and greasiness when cleaning with pine. Pine is recommended for use in bathroom and oven cleaning where grout may be present, ultimately the fresh scent and anti-septic qualities leave even hard to clean surfaces germ free and pleasantly scented. It follows that the use of pine in laundry washing is also a recommended application as the stiff, though fresh essence leaves fabrics crisp and aromatically pleasing.

Bathroom and Kitchen Mould

Another age old remedy for cleaning is the use of clove oil. When used as an oil clove can be very useful when cleaning most areas of the house from the kitchen to bathrooms to bedrooms and hallways. Clove is known to be a very useful in the removal of mould and grout from bathrooms and from the kitchen.

Its application can be used by the addition of oils into a cleaning spray. Although the best method of use when cleaning with clove is in the form of a scrub, this is due to the potent nature of clove and its robust properties. Especially useful when dealing with tough stains, mould and mildew, clove scrub is preferred as it can be centralized to the necessary area, whereas a spray is more dispersed a scrub can be applied more specifically to areas of difficulty.

Clove has a strong essence, which is ideal to use when dealing with carpet stains. The ratio is generally ½ teaspoon per 1 litre of water, this should be sprayed onto the stain and allowed to soak for overnight before adding salt to assist in evaporation, then wiping or vacuuming away the remnants. On top of its wide variety of uses, clove is also high in antiviral and antiseptic qualities while also creating a delightful aroma when used in cleaning or even when used simply for its aromatic properties. An important side note when dealing with clove is the potential for skin irritation if over exposed, this is a minor issue though it does lead to the recommendation of using gloves when cleaning with clove, especially in the form of paste. It is also subsequently important to ensure that once cleaning is complete any remnants are wiped from the area, furthermore this advice should be heeded with just about any cleaning product natural or synthetic.

Finally, it is true that there are many, many more alternative uses and ingredients when using aromatherapy in the home, though it is hoped that these ideas above have not only shown you the ease with which aromatherapy can be used around the home but also the benefits of doing so.

It is important to remember that what can be achieved through synthetic cleaning products can be done just as well, if not better through the use of natural products. When coupled with the fact that you can personalize aromatic products to your preferences, it seems a good reason to at least try the natural alternative of aromatherapy.

Moreover it should be made clear that by no means are the above remedies the only options, there are countless combinations of oils and herbs that can aid in countless spheres of life. Aromatherapy is not only scented candles and incense it is an avenue to creating all natural alternatives that reap the same results as store bought remedies or cleaning products. From insomnia to bathroom grout and mildew there is a remedy for everything when using aromatic therapies and remedies in everyday life.

SUMMARY

Aromatherapy is gradually taking over from other forms of medicines and is becoming increasingly popular amongst people who seek cheaper and natural forms of these medicines. The best part about aromatherapy is that it can be offered as a complementary therapy or, more controversially, as form of alternative medicine. Complementary therapy can be offered alongside standard treatment, with alternative medicine offered instead of conventional treatments, conventional treatments being often scientifically proven. It is a natural, non-invasive method designed to affect the whole person not just the symptom or disease and to assist the body's natural ability to balance, regulate, heal and maintain itself through the correct use of essential oils.

It's even known that aromatherapy is dominating the health market and is widely and cheaply available, as one can always make the oil in its natural form as against the chemically induced medicines with expiry dates or the oils that are available pre-made which could be costly due to branding. It's common to have the prices hiked due to either quality or the oils being labeled as 'luxury or premium' when actually they don't differ from oils that you can buy in health stores individually or in bulk. So you can easily make the recipes from the comfort of your own home that you'd otherwise have to buy for double the price if it was pre-made by a brand.

Even though essential oils have been used for centuries, few studies have actually looked into the safety and effectiveness of aromatherapy in people. Scientific evidence is lacking and there are some concerns about the safety and quality of certain essential oils, although that doesn't mean they aren't effective or beneficial, especially since they have been used for a very long time. But, more research is needed before aromatherapy becomes a widely accepted alternative remedy.

So, when you're looking into the purchase or use of essential oils, it would be good to become educated on what these oils would be good for, as some of these were stated in the book. This would help to avoid any complications or bad advice that could otherwise lead to negative effects like rashes, especially if you might be allergic to any ingredients, which would not be intended by the author of the book. Getting proper guidance first hand is always useful for reaping the maximum benefits of Aromatherapy.

Thus concludes our wonderful journey into the world of Aromatherapy. I hope you had a knowledgeable and enlightening time whilst reading this book and gaining the insight into aromatherapy. I also hope that you have learned that there is more than one way to use aromatherapy and many more to yet be mentioned.

Relax and enjoy your wellness in Aromatherapy.

ABOUT THE AUTHOR

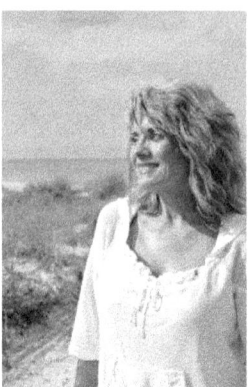

Ruth Logan has been fascinated with Personal Development, Health, and Wellbeing for just over 30 years now. She's particularly passionate about Eastern Philosophy, and the Science behind Wellbeing. Her aim is to share the great benefits of Eastern Philosophy to the unaware in modern society.

Ruth is an avid reader and can't resist learning new information on how we can all better ourselves. Over the last couple of years she's started freelance writing and more recently taken the step to releasing her on work.

In her books, Ruth provides action plans and advice on how to incorporate learning points into 'real life' in a concise yet informative manner.

When not reading or writing, Ruth enjoys walking her dog, cooking and travel.

MORE BOOKS BY RUTH LOGAN

If you enjoyed reading **"Aromatherapy"**, you may like these other books from Ruth Logan.

Beauty Bath – How to Create a Professional Quality Home Spa for Relaxation and Pure Indulgence

Gratitude – 7 Simple Steps To Becoming More Grateful In 7 Days

Healing – 7 Ways To Heal Your Body in 7 Days

Learning – 7 Steps To Increasing Your Learning Your Learning Potential In 7 Days

Limiting Beliefs – 7 Ways To Stop Limiting Beliefs In 7 Days